FOOD GIRL

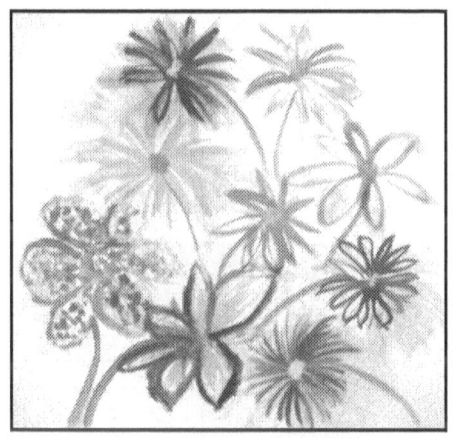

DONNA REGA

Note for Librarians: A cataloguing record for this book is available from Library and Archives
Canada at www.collectionscanada.ca/amicus/index-e.html
ISBN 1-4251-0219-0

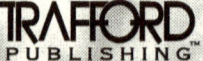

PUBLISHING

Offices in Canada, USA, Ireland and UK

Book sales for North America and international:
Trafford Publishing, 6E–2333 Government St.,
Victoria, BC V8T 4P4 CANADA
phone 250 383 6864 (toll-free 1 888 232 4444)
fax 250 383 6804; email to orders@trafford.com
Book sales in Europe:
Trafford Publishing (UK) Limited, 9 Park End Street, 2nd Floor
Oxford, UK OX1 1HH UNITED KINGDOM
phone 44 (0)1865 722 113 (local rate 0845 230 9601)
facsimile 44 (0)1865 722 868; info.uk@trafford.com
Order online at:
trafford.com/06-1976

10 9 8 7 6 5 4 3

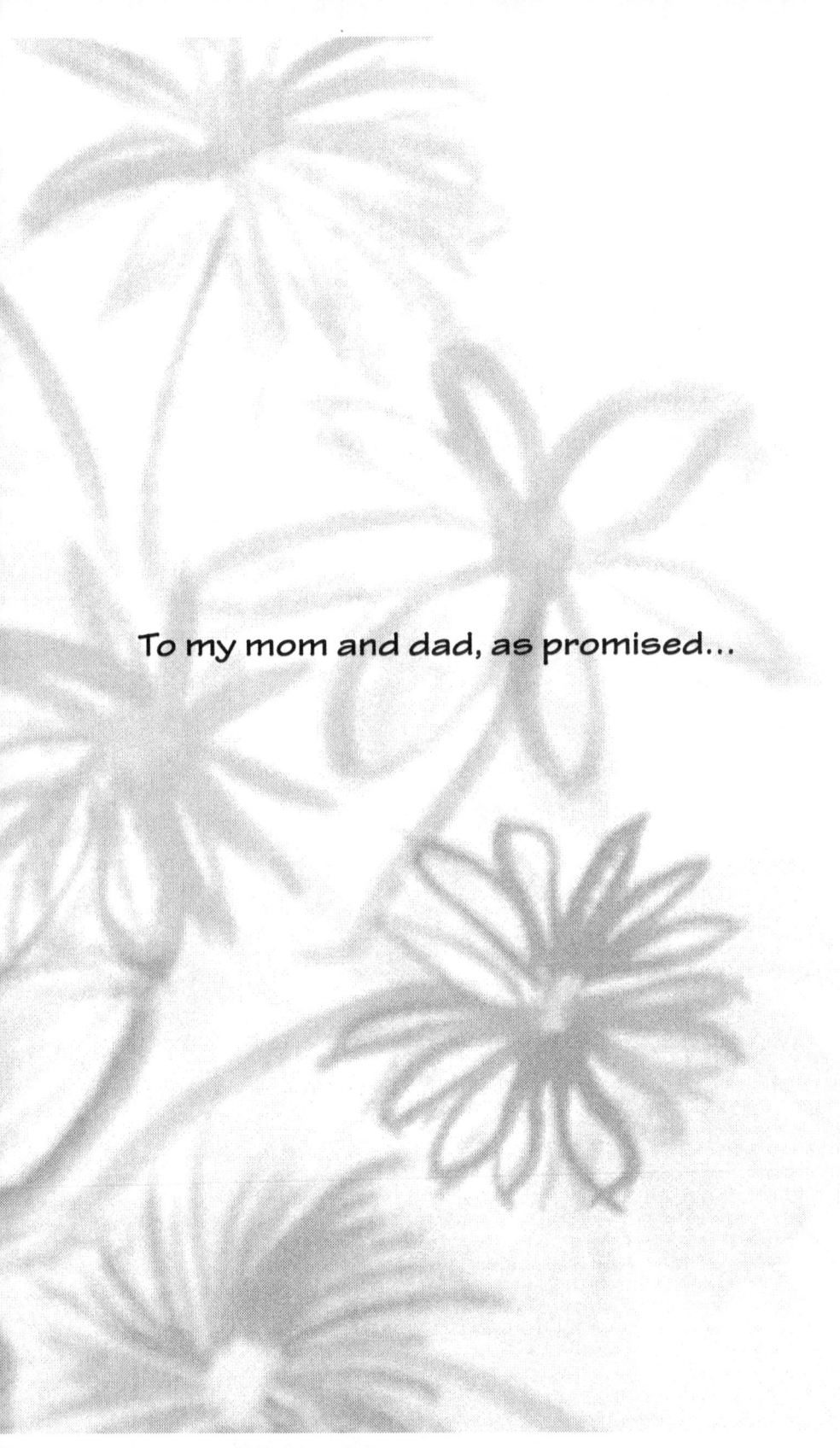

To my mom and dad, as promised...

TABLE OF CONTENTS

BREAD STICKS AND PROSCIUTTO

¼ lb. Prosciutto
10 Sesame Seeded Bread Sticks

Take a slice of prosciutto and rip it in half lengthwise. Use one half and wrap it around a bread stick. Continue until all have been arranged. Serve standing in a glass.

BREAD/FIG/WALNUT

1 Slice Crusty Bread
2 Fresh Figs
4 Walnut Pieces

Cut the slice of crusty bread into 4 sections. Cut the figs
in half. Place one section of bread on a plate, top with one
half of a fig and put the walnut on top of the fig. Continue
until all ingredients are finished. Serve.

_____

_____

_____

FANCY OLIVE OIL DIP

¼ c. Olive Oil
1 tsp. Oregano
1 tsp. Grated Reggiano Parminaggio Cheese
1 tsp. Red Pepper Flakes
1 tsp. Basil
1 loaf Crusty Italian Bread

In a dish, place olive oil, oregano, grated cheese, red pepper flakes and basil. Slice the crusty Italian bread. Dip away.

SHRIMP COCKTAIL

1 doz. Shrimp
1 tsp. Tabasco Sauce
4 T. Ketchup
3 Leaves of Lettuce
1 tsp. White Vinegar
½ Lemon

Wash and devain shrimp. Leave tails on. Bring a pot of water to a boil. Add vinegar and shrimp. Shrimp are cooked when they turn pink and white. Drain and rinse with cold water. Place in the refrigerator until cold. In a small bowl, mix Tabasco sauce, juice of the lemon and ketchup. Wash and dry lettuce. Place lettuce on a platter. Arrange shrimp on top of the lettuce. Put sauce in a small bowl and place in the center of platter. Serve chilled.

FIZZIN PINA COLADA SMOOTHIE

1 6oz. Pineapple Coconut Yogurt
1 slice Pineapple
1 tsp. Sugar
4 Ice Cubes
½ c. Plain Seltzer

Place yogurt, pineapple, sugar in a blender. Mix until smooth. Add ice. Blend until smooth. Add seltzer and pulse a couple times. Serve in a tall glass with a straw.

FRESH HOMEMADE LEMONADE

3 lg. Lemons
¼ c. Sugar
4 c. Water
1 c. Ice

Slice lemons in half and squeeze juice in a pitcher. Add sugar and water. Stir until sugar has dissolved. Add ice and serve.

LEMON AND LIMEADE

2 Lemons
2 Limes
¼ c. Sugar
4 c. Water
1 c. Ice

Slice lemons and limes, squeeze juice into a pitcher. Add sugar and water. Stir until sugar dissolves. Add ice and serve.

LEMON AND ORANGEADE

2 Oranges
2 Lemons
¼ c. Sugar
6 c. Water
1 c. Ice

Slice oranges and lemons in half and squeeze juice into a pitcher. Add sugar and water. Stir until sugar dissolves. Add ice and serve.

_____

_____

_____

_____

ORANGE BANANA SMOOTHIE

½ c. Orange Juice
½ Banana
½ c. Vanilla Yogurt
2 Ice Cubes
2 T. Water

In a blender, add orange juice, banana, yogurt, ice cubes, and water. Blend until smooth. Serve.

LOL ADE (LEMON/ORANGE/LIME)

1 Lemon
1 Lime
2 Oranges
¼ c. Sugar
6 c. Water
1 c. Ice

Slice lemon, lime, oranges in half and squeeze juice into a pitcher. Add sugar and water. Stir until sugar dissolves. Add ice and serve.

STRAWBERRY SMOOTHIE

7 Strawberries
1 tsp. Sugar
1 6oz Vanilla Yogurt
3 Ice Cubes

Wash and hull strawberries. Place strawberries, sugar, and yogurt in a blender. Mix until well blended. Add ice cubes and pulse until smooth. Serve.

CHICKEN SOUP

3 Chicken Cutlets
3 stalks Celery sliced
3 Carrots sliced
½ tsp. Peppercorns
½ c. Tube Macaroni (or any small shape pasta)
Pinch Salt
Grated Cheese

Wash and dry chicken cutlets. Bring 5 cups of water to a boil. Add chicken to boiling water. Bring to a second boil. Remove chicken and let cool. In the same pot the chicken came out of add celery, carrots, peppercorns, and salt. Bring to a third boil. Shred chicken. Add macaroni and chicken. Cook until macaroni has come to desired tenderness. Spoon into plate and top with grated cheese. Serve.

ESCAROLE AND BEANS SOUP

1 head Escarole
3 T. Olive Oil
2 cloves Garlic peeled
1 15oz. can Small White Beans strained
½ c. Chicken Stock
Pinch Salt
Hard (Stale) Whole Wheat Bread Biscuits
Grated Cheese

Wash and tear escarole. In a saucepan, add olive oil and garlic cloves. Let that infuse for a minute. Add escarole, white beans, chicken stock, and salt. Cover the saucepan. Bring to a simmer. Let simmer until escarole wilts and becomes soft. Stir occasionally. Put a piece of hard bread in a dish and add a large spoonful of escarole and beans on top it. Add some grated cheese. Serve.

ONE POT ESCAROLE
AND CHICKEN SOUP

3 Chicken Cutlets
1 bunch Escarole
2 gloves Garlic peeled
4 c. Chicken Stock
Grated Cheese

Wash and cut escarole. In a saucepan, add olive oil, and garlic. Infuse for a couple of minutes. Add escarole and simmer until it wilts. Add chicken stock. Bring to a boil. To the same saucepan, add chicken cutlets. Bring to a second boil. Remove chicken cutlets. Let cool and shred. Add shredded chicken to pot. Bring to a third boil. Spoon into plate and top with a pinch of grated cheese. Serve.

LENTIL SOUP

1 c. Lentils
2 T. Olive Oil
4 slices Deli Ham cut into small pieces
½ Onion chopped
1 stalk Celery chopped
1 clove Garlic
1 c. Chicken Broth
2 c. Water
Salt and Pepper

Sort and rinse lentils. In a saucepan, add oil, ham, celery, onion, and garlic. Cook until celery and onion are soft. Add lentils, chicken broth, salt, pepper, and water. Bring to a boil. Reduce heat. Cover and simmer until lentils are tender and soup gets thick. Add more water if necessary. Serve.

MEATBALL ESCAROLE SOUP

7 c. Chicken Broth
2 cloves Garlic
1 lb. Chop Meat
¼ c. Grated Cheese
1 head Escarole

Put chicken broth in a large pot and bring to a boil. Wash and cut escarole. Add escarole and garlic to boiling chicken broth. Bring to a second boil. In the meantime, in a bowl mix chop meat and grated cheese. Form into tiny meatballs. Add meatballs into pot. Bring to a third boil. Simmer for 5 minutes and serve with bread.

TURKEY SOUP

2 slices Turkey cutlets
1 Carrot sliced
1 stalk Celery sliced
¼ c. Small Pasta
Salt and Pepper

Bring a pot of water to a boil. Add turkey. Bring to a second boil. Let boil for 5 minutes. Take turkey cutlets out of water. Let cool. Shred. Into same water, add carrots, celery, salt, and pepper. Cook until carrots and celery are almost tender. Add pasta and shredded turkey. Bring to a third boil. Cook for 10 additional minutes or until pasta is to desired tenderness. Serve.

COLE SLAW

½ c. Mayonnaise
2 T. White Vinegar
2 T. Milk
½ tsp. Sugar
2 T. Celery Seed
4 oz. sliced Green Cabbage
4 oz. sliced Red Cabbage

In a bowl mix mayo, vinegar, milk, sugar, and celery seed. Stir in green and red cabbage. Refrigerate for 2 hours and serve.

SPINACH SALAD

2 c. Fresh Spinach
½ Red Onion
1 Hard Boiled Egg shelled
1 Tomatoe
2 T. Olive Oil
1 T. Vinegar
Pinch Salt and Pepper

Wash spinach. Slice onion, tomatoe, and hard boiled egg. In a bowl place spinach, onion, sliced hard boiled egg, tomatoe, oil, vinegar, salt, and pepper. Toss and serve.

TOMATOE SALAD

1 lg. Tomatoe
2 cloves Garlic
1 tsp. Oregano
2 T. Olive Oil
Salt

Wash and slice tomatoe. Place in a large flat dish so that the slices are a single layer. Peel and slice garlic. Place sliced garlic on top of sliced tomatoe. Sprinkle with oregano, salt, and olive oil. Serve room temperature.

BLUE CHEESE AND TOMATOE SALAD

2 Tomatoes
¼ c. Blue Cheese crumbled
2 T. Italian Salad Dressing

Wash and slice tomatoes. In a dish add sliced tomatoes, blue cheese and Italian salad dressing. Toss and serve.

TUNA FISH SALAD

1 can Solid White Tuna in Water
1 tsp. Balsamic Vinegar
1 T. Mayonnaise

Wash tuna under cold water. Drain. In a bowl, add tuna, vinegar, and mayonnaise. Mash and mix well. Serve.

WEDGES OF LETTUCE

1 head Iceberg Lettuce
¼ lb. Blue Cheese
4 Plum Tomatoes
1 Seedless Cucumber
1 8oz. bottle Italian Salad Dressing

Wash and cut lettuce into 4 wedges. Wash and cut tomatoes, and cucumber into chunks. On a large flat plate, place wedges of lettuce, a pile of tomatoes, a separate pile of cucumbers and another pile of blue cheese. Pour salad dressing on top of lettuce, tomatoes, cucumbers, and blue cheese. Serve.

SPECIAL BROCCOLI

1 bunch Broccoli
1 clove Garlic peeled
½ Lemon
2 T. Olive Oil
Salt to taste

Bring a pot of water to boil. Add broccoli. Boil for 5 minutes.
Strain. Place broccoli in a bowl. Squeeze lemon over broccoli.
Add olive oil, garlic, and salt. Toss. Serve.

DELICIOUS PEAS

1 pkg. Frozen Peas
1 sm. Onion
1 tsp. Black Pepper
¼ c. Water

Chop onion. In a pot, add frozen peas, onion, black pepper, and water. Bring to a boil. Simmer for 5 minutes. Serve.

GARLIC POTATOE CROQUETS

5 lbs. Potatoes
3 Eggs
1 c. Plain Bread Crumbs
1 c. Vegetable Oil
3 cloves Garlic peeled
Salt and Pepper

Wash and peel potatoes. Cut into chunks. In a pot, add water to cover potatoes. Bring to a boil. Potatoes are done when fork goes through potatoe chunk easily. Strain. Mash. Wait until potatoes cool. In a skillet with one tablespoon of vegetable oil sauté garlic cloves until golden and soft. Strain. Mash. Add garlic, eggs, salt, and pepper to potatoe mash. Take tablespoonfuls of potatoe mash and shape into strips. Keep cold. Place bread crumbs in a dish. Roll and coat potatoe strips into bread crumbs. Preheat vegetable oil. Place strips of coated potatoes into preheated oil. Turn once. They are done when golden brown. Serve hot or cold.

_____

_____

_____

_____

HOT GREEN ITALIAN PEPPERS

1 lb. Hot Long Green Peppers
5 cloves Garlic peeled
¼ c. Olive Oil
Salt to taste

Wash peppers, dry and trim stems. In a pan, under low heat, warm olive oil. Add garlic. Wait until garlic is golden brown. Add peppers and cover pan. Simmer for half an hour or until the peppers wilt. Transfer to a bowl and add a pinch of salt. Serve with crusty bread.

ROASTED RED/GREEN/ YELLOW PEPPERS

9 Peppers assorted colors
¼ c. Olive Oil
1 head Garlic peeled and chopped

Wash and dry peppers. Place on a cookie sheet. Preheat broiler. Place cookie sheet with peppers under the broiler. Set timer for 3 minutes. Check to see if the tops of peppers turn a dark color. If not, set the timer for another 3 minutes. If they do turn a dark color, then turn the peppers onto the next side and set the timer for another 3 minutes. Repeat until the whole pepper is a dark color. Take pepper out of the broiler and cool. Over a bowl, peel the skin from each pepper allowing any liquid to fall into bowl. Discard the seeds. Rip pepper into strips. Add olive oil, and garlic. Serve with crusty bread.

STEAMED POTATOES

5 lbs. Potatoes
1 large Onion peeled and sliced
Salt and Pepper to taste
1 c. Water

Preheat oven to 350 degrees. Wash, peel and slice potatoes. Place potatoes, onion, salt, pepper, water in a baking dish. Cover with aluminum foil. Bake in oven for 1 hour or until desired tenderness. Check every 20 minutes if additional water is needed. Serve.

S.P.O.C.T. SALAD

1 lb. String Beans cooked
1 Potatoe boiled
½ sm. Red Onion
1 stalk Celery
1 Tomatoe
½ tsp. Oregano
3 T. Olive Oil
Salt to taste
2 Pc. Hard Wheat Bread

Slice potatoe, tomatoe, celery, and onion. Place in a bowl with string beans. Add oregano, salt, and olive oil. Toss. Run the hard wheat bread under water and serve together.

STRING BEAN SALAD

1 lb. String Beans
2 cloves Garlic peeled
½ tsp. Oregano
Salt to taste
1 T. Olive Oil
1 tsp. Vinegar

Cut off stems of string beans. Bring 4 cups of water to a boil. Place string beans into boiling water. Let them come to a second boil. Pinch one of the string beans to see if done to desired tenderness. Strain and place under cold water. Strain. In a bowl, add string beans, garlic, oregano, salt, olive oil, and vinegar. Toss and serve.

STRING BEANS AND BREAD CRUMBS

1 LB. String Beans
½ stick Butter
¼ c. Plain Bread Crumbs
1 clove Garlic peeled and chopped

Wash and trim ends from string beans. Bring a pot of water to a boil and place string beans into boiling water. Bring to a second boil. Cook to desired tenderness. Strain. Preheat oven to 350 degrees. In a baking dish, place string beans, butter, and garlic. Allow the butter to melt about 3 minutes. Take the baking dish out of the oven and add the bread crumbs. Toss. Place back in the oven for 3 minutes so that the bread crumbs brown. Serve.

STRING BEANS AND GARLIC

1 lb. String Beans cooked
3 cloves Garlic peeled and chopped
¼ c. Olive Oil
Salt to taste

In a pan place olive oil and garlic under low heat. Sauté for 2 minutes. In a bowl, place string beans, salt, heated olive oil and garlic. Toss. Serve.

STRING BEANS AND POTATOE SALAD

1 lb. String Beans
2 Potatoes
1 clove Garlic peeled
¼ c. Olive Oil
Salt to taste

Peel potatoes and cut into small pieces. Wash and trim ends off of string beans. Place potatoes into a pot of water and bring to a boil. All to cook for 5 minutes then add string beans into same pot as the potatoes. Bring to a third boil. Cook to desired tenderness. Once done, strain. In a bowl, add potatoes, string beans, garlic, salt, and olive oil. Serve.

STUFFED ARTICHOKES

3 Artichokes
½ c. Bread Crumbs
¼ c. Parsley chopped
2 cloves Garlic peeled and chopped
¼ c. Grated Parmigiana Cheese
Stems of Artichokes peeled and chopped
2 env. Powder Chicken Broth
1 c. Water
2 T. Olive Oil
Crusty Bread

Cut stems from the bottom of artichokes. Chop and put into a large bowl. Rinse artichokes. Slam artichoke top side down to open artichoke. Cut tips of leaves on artichokes. Drain upside down. In the same bowl with the chopped artichoke stems, add bread crumbs, parsley, garlic, and grated cheese. Mix with spoon until blended. Separate and open leaves with one hand and spoon mixture into artichoke with the other hand. Place in a pot. Repeat with the other artichokes. Make sure all the artichokes touch in the pot so that they do not fall. In a bowl, mix powder chicken broth and water. Add to pot with the stuffed artichokes. Drizzle olive oil. Cover and bring to a boil. Lower heat to a simmer. Cook 2 hours. Check every half hour to see if you need to add more liquid. Serve with crusty bread.

A LITTLE OF EVERYTHING

1 T. Olive Oil
4 cloves Garlic peeled
1 sm. Onion peeled
1 sm. Zucchini
4 Mushrooms
2 pcs. Roasted Peppers
1 sm. Eggplant
1 Tomatoe
3 Chicken Cutlets
Salt to taste

Wash and chop veggies. Heat skillet, add olive oil, garlic, and onion. Sauté on low heat until onion begins to turn soft. Add zucchini, mushrooms, roasted peppers, eggplant, tomatoes, chicken and salt. Cover and simmer for 15 minutes. Check to see if veggies and chicken are done to desired tenderness. Serve.

BACCALA ITALIAN STYLE

1 pc. Dried Baccala
1 Potatoe peeled and cut into chunks
pinch Red Pepper Flakes
pinch Oregano
8 oz. Water

Soak baccala for 3 days. Change water each day. After third day, in a pot add baccala, red pepper flakes, oregano, water, and potatoes. Bring to a boil. Let cook for 15 minutes or until the baccala falls apart or skin falls off. Serve hot.

BROCCOLI RABE/SAUSAGE/
HARD BREAD

1 lb. Broccoli Rabe
4 Sausage links
Olive Oil
2 Pieces Hard Bread

Bring a pot of water to boil. In the meantime, wash and cut
ends off of broccoli rabe. When water comes to a boil, place
broccoli rabe into pot. Let it come to a second boil. Cook
for about 10 minutes. Strain and place under cold water
to keep color. This will also take the bitterness out of the
broccoli rabe. Squeeze the water out of the broccoli rabe.
Take sausage out of casing and place in a skillet, cook until
brown. Run hard bread under water. In the same skillet as
the sausage, add broccoli rabe, moistened bread. Remove
from heat and add olive oil. Toss. Serve warm.

BROCCOLI RABE/SAUSAGE/POTATOES

1 lb. Broccoli Rabe
4 Sausage links
2 T. Olive Oil
2 Potatoes

Wash and cut ends of broccoli rabe. Bring a pot of water to a boil. Add broccoli rabe to boiling water. Cook until done to desired tenderness. Strain. Run under cold water. Squeeze excess water out of broccoli rabe. Poke holes in potatoes and place in a microwave for 3 minutes. Rotate potatoes and repeat until soft to the touch. Slice potatoes. Place olive oil in a skillet. Take sausage out of casing and add to olive oil. Cook until golden brown. Add sliced potatoes and broccoli rabe. Once the broccoli rabe is warm usually 2 minutes serve.

BROILED FLOUNDER

2 pcs. Flounder
2 T. Olive Oil
1 tsp. Oregano
1 clove Garlic peeled and chopped
1 tsp. Basil
1 tsp. Parsley
1 Lemon
3 T. Bread Crumbs
Salt and Pepper to taste

Wash and dry flounder. Preheat broiler. In a baking dish, drizzle one tablespoon olive oil and place flounder on top of it. Sprinkle oregano, basil, garlic, parsley, juice of lemon, bread crumbs, salt, pepper and remainder tablespoon of olive oil. Place in broiler for 10-15 minutes. Serve.

CHICKEN STRIPS

3 Chicken Cutlets
2 Eggs
1 tsp. Milk
1 c. Plain Bread Crumbs
Salt and Pepper to taste
½ c. Vegetable Oil

In a bowl, beat eggs, milk, salt, and pepper. Set aside. Place bread crumbs in another dish. Place vegetable oil in a skillet to heat. Wash and dry chicken cutlets. Cut into strips. Dip chicken strips into egg mixture. Then dip into bread crumbs. Make sure to cover entire chicken strips with egg mixture and bread crumbs. Place into heated vegetable oil. Turn after 3-5 minutes. Place paper towels on a dish. Once chicken strips are golden brown take out of the oil. Place onto dish with paper towels to drain excess oil. Serve.

SIMPLE EGG SALAD

2 Eggs
1 tsp. Mayonnaise
2 Bread Rolls

Place two eggs into a pot of cold water and bring to a boil.
Boil for 7 minutes. Strain. Peel shells from eggs. Mash eggs
in a bowl. Add mayonnaise and mix. Slice rolls lengthwise in
half. Divide egg salad in half. Spoon half of the egg salad on
each roll. Serve.

FRENCH TOAST SANDWICH

2 slices Bread
2 slices Deli Ham
2 slices Munster Cheese
¼ c. Maple Syrup
1 Egg
1 T. Butter

Preheat stovetop grill. Place slices of ham and cheese in between two slices of bread. Beat egg. Dip sandwich into egg. Slide butter all over grill to cover area where sandwich will be placed. Place sandwich on hot grill at least 1-2 minutes on each side. Serve with maple syrup.

FRENCH TOAST SUPREME

3 Eggs
¼ c. Milk
1 dash Cinnamon
1 tsp. Vanilla
2 tsp. grated Orange peel
3 Strawberries sliced
2 Bananas sliced
1 dash Sugar
½ c. Orange Juice
7 slices Bread
1 T. Butter

Preheat stovetop grill. Mix eggs, milk, cinnamon, vanilla, one teaspoon grated orange peel, and ¼ cup of the orange juice until well blended. Slide butter all over grill to cover area where bread will be placed. Dip slices of bread into mixture and place onto grill. Grill for 2 minutes on each side. In a bowl, mix strawberries, bananas, 1 teaspoon grated orange peel, sugar, and ¼ cup of orange juice. Place fruit mixture on top of cooked French toast and serve.

GRILLED SANDWICH

2 slices Ham
2 slices Munster Cheese
2 slices Bread
3 slices Tomatoes
1 tsp. Olive Oil

Preheat stovetop grill. Place ham, cheese, and tomatoe slices in between two slices of bread. Smear olive oil on outside slices of sandwich. Place onto the hot grill for 2 minutes on each side. Serve.

HOMEMADE GNOCCHI

¼ c. Water
1 c. Flour
1 tsp. Olive Oil
1 Baked Potatoe

In a bowl, mash baked potatoe and add flour, water, and olive oil. Mix and form into a ball. Add more water if needed. If the dough is too sticky add some flour. Roll ball into a log. Cut off ¼ inch stubs and run fork over to create lines on it. Bring a pot of water to a boil. Drop gnocchi into boiling water for 1 minute. When gnocchi surface to the top of water, they are done. Strain. Serve with your favorite sauce.

LEFTOVER CHICKEN DISH

½ c. Rice
1 c. Chicken Stock
¼ c. Mixed Nuts
½ c. Shredded Leftover Chicken
Salt and Pepper to taste

Cook rice according to directions on package using chicken stock instead of water. Last 2 minutes of cooking time add nuts and shredded chicken. Serve.

LEFTOVER TURKEY SANDWICH

¼ lb. Leftover Turkey
1 slice Cranberry Jelly
1 Roll toasted
2 T. Stuffing

Place turkey, cranberry sauce and stuffing on roll. Serve.

LENTIL SALAD

5 T. Olive Oil
1 ¼ c. Lentils
Salt and Pepper to taste
3 ½ c. Chicken Stock
1 Bay Leaf
½ c. Carrots
½ c. Zucchini
½ c. Onion
½ c. Celery
1 clove Garlic peeled
1 T. Balsamic Vinegar

Wash and dice carrots, zucchini, onion, and celery. In a saucepan, put 2 tablespoons of olive oil, lentils, garlic, salt and pepper. Let brown for 2 minutes. Add chicken stock and bay leaf. Bring to a boil. Simmer for 30 minutes. In another skillet, add carrots, zucchini, onion, celery, and 2 tablespoons of olive oil. Cook for 10 minutes or until tender. When lentils are tender, drain but reserve ½ cup of liquid. Return lentils and liquid to skillet with vegetables and bring to a simmer. Remove from heat. Remove bay leaf. Stir in balsamic vinegar and last tablespoon of olive oil. Serve.

MACARONI/ESCAROLE/BEANS

1 bunch Escarole
3 T. Olive Oil
2 cloves Garlic peeled
1 15oz. c. Small White Beans strained
1 c. Chicken Stock
½ c. Elbow Macaroni
1 pinch Salt
Grated Cheese

Wash and cut escarole. In a heated saucepan, add olive oil, and garlic cloves. Keep on low heat for a minute. Add escarole, white beans, chicken stock, and salt. Bring to a simmer until escarole wilts. In the meantime, bring another pot of water to a boil. Add macaroni. Cook to desired tenderness. Save half a cup of the water from the macaroni. Strain the remaining water. Add the half cup of macaroni water, and macaroni to the saucepan with the escarole and beans. Stir. Place a spoonful of escarole, beans, and macaroni in a dish. Add grated cheese on top. Serve.

MEATBALLS AND TOMATOE SAUCE

3 T. Olive Oil
9 cloves Garlic peeled
1 Onion
2 28oz. cans Tomatoes
1 sm. Can Tomatoe Paste
2 T. Oregano
2 T. Basil

5 links Sausage
1 lb. Chopped Beef
2 eggs
1 tsp. Parsley Flakes
1 T. Grated Parmigiana Cheese
¼ c. Plain Bread Crumbs
Salt and Pepper to taste

Peel and chop onion. In a skillet add olive oil, onion, seven garlic cloves, and sausage. Cook sausage through about 10-15 minutes until golden brown. Open cans of tomatoes. In a large pot, add tomatoes, tomatoe paste, oregano, basil, and salt. Cover and bring to a boil. Once sausage is done place into pot with tomatoes. In a bowl, add chopped beef, parsley flakes, grated cheese, salt, pepper, two chopped cloves garlic, bread crumbs, and eggs. Mix with hands until well blended. If mixture is to sticky add a little more bread crumbs. Form into small balls. Place into same skillet as sausage. Turn meatballs until golden brown. When meatballs are done, place into pot with tomatoes. After all sausage and meatballs are finished pour olive oil, garlic and onions from the skillet into pot of tomatoes. Cover pot with tomatoes and keep flame at its' lowest. Let simmer for 2 hours. Serve sauce with meatballs or make small portions of meatballs and sauce and place in freezer. Can also serve with your favorite pasta. Cook pasta according to directions on package. Strain and add sauce on top of pasta. Serve.

ANNA'S TOMATOE SANDWICH

1 sliced Tomatoe
1 clove Garlic peeled and chopped
1 pinch Salt
1 pinch Oregano
1 splash Olive Oil
1 sm. roll Crusty Bread

Open bread in form of a well with hands. Place tomatoes on bottom. Add garlic, salt, oregano, and olive oil. Serve.

BENNY'S BACCALA

1 pc. Baccala
3 tomatoes washed
1 clove Garlic peeled
1 Potatoe peeled
2 stalks Celery
1 Onion peeled
1 pinch Salt
2 T. Olive Oil

Soak baccala for 3 days. Change water every day. In a skillet, add olive oil, and garlic. Cook under low heat until garlic is golden. Chop potatoe, celery, tomatoes, and onion. Add potatoe, celery, onion, baccala, and tomatoes to skillet and bring to a simmer. Add pinch of salt. Let simmer until baccala falls apart or skin falls off. Serve.

OPEN FACED SANDWICH

8 oz. Brown Gravy
½ lb. Sliced Deli Roast Beef
½ loaf White Bread

Warm gravy in a pan. Bring to a slight simmer. Stirring constantly. Add roast beef slices, one at a time until all slices are covered with gravy. It is ready once pink on roast beef slices turn brown. In a dish, place one slice of white bread and spoon a couple slices of roast beef with gravy on top. Serve.

ORANGE FLAVORED PANCAKES

1 c. Pancake Mix
¾ c. Milk
1 Egg
1 tsp. Oil
1 Orange
¼ c. Syrup
1 tsp. Butter

Preheat stovetop grill. In a bowl mix pancake mix, milk, egg, oil, juice and zest of orange.
Rub butter on stovetop grill. Drop spoonfuls of batter onto grill. Flip when bubbles form. Serve with syrup. Makes approximately 10 pancakes.

PASTA AND STRING BEANS

½ lb. Pasta
½ lb. Green Beans chopped
1 Tomatoe chopped
2 cloves Garlic peeled and chopped
1 tsp. Oregano
2 T. Olive Oil
2 T. Grated Cheese

Wash and trim ends from string beans. Cook pasta according to directions on package. Add string beans half way through cooking time of pasta. Take a spoonful of the water from the pasta and reserve. Strain pasta and string beans. In a pot add reserved pasta water, olive oil, garlic, oregano, tomatoes and bring to a simmer. Continue to simmer for at least 5 minutes. Add pasta, string beans, and grated cheese. Serve.

PASTA AND PEAS

½ lb. Pasta
¼ c. Peas
½ Onion peeled and chopped
1 Tomatoe diced
2 cloves Garlic peeled and chopped
1 tsp. Oregano
2 T. Olive Oil
2 T. Grated Cheese

Cook pasta according to directions on package. The last minute add peas. Strain. In a pan, add olive oil, garlic, onion, tomatoes, and oregano. Cook until onions are soft. Add pasta and peas. Sprinkle with grated cheese. Serve.

PASTA AND BEANS

1 can Small White Beans
1 Tomatoe
2 cloves garlic peeled
1 stalk celery with leaves chopped
1 tsp. Oregano
2 T. Olive Oil
½ lb. Pasta

In a pot add 5 cups of water, tomatoe, garlic, celery, oregano, and olive oil. Bring to a boil and add pasta. Let pasta cook about 8-10 minutes and add beans. Simmer for another 3 minutes. Serve.

PEPPERS AND EGGS

1-2 piece/s Roasted Red Pepper
1-2 piece/s Roasted Green Pepper
3 Eggs
¼ c. Cheddar Cheese shredded
1 tsp. Milk
1 Soft Tortilla
1 tsp. Olive Oil
Salt and Pepper to taste

In a bowl beat eggs, milk, salt, and pepper. Place olive oil in a skillet and add egg mixture. Keep on low heat. With a fork keep mixing egg mixture until cooked. Heat another pan large enough to fit the tortilla so that it lays flat. Heat up each side of tortilla. A minute on each side. Keep on low heat. Once tortilla has been turned to heat the second side, add cheddar cheese and spoonful of cooked eggs to cover tortilla. Add the roasted peppers on top of the eggs. Carefully remove and cut into four pieces. Serve.

POT ROAST

1 5lb. Rump Bottom Round Beef Roast
2 Carrots
1 Onion peeled
2 stalks Celery
2 T. Parsley
2 c. Water

In a pot add rump roast, carrots, onion, celery, parsley, and water. Cover the pot and cook on medium heat for 2 hours. Every half hour check the water level. If the water level drops add more water. Once the two hours pass turn the heat off and let it sit for a half hour. Slice and serve.

QUICK STEAK

1 ½ lb. T-Bone Steak
2 cloves Garlic peeled and sliced
Salt and Pepper to taste

Preheat broiler. On a cookie sheet place slices of garlic on top and bottom of steak. Sprinkle with salt and pepper. Put into broiler for 5 minutes on each side or to desired tenderness. Serve.

QUICK STUFFING AND CHICKEN

1 pkg. Stuffing Mix
3 Chicken Cutlets
1 T. Olive Oil
1 sm. Onion

Cook stuffing according to directions. In a skillet add olive oil and onion. Cook for 2 minutes on low heat. Wash and dry chicken cutlets. Cut chicken cutlets into chunks. Add to skillet. Cover and simmer for 10 minutes. Once cooked through add stuffing and toss. Serve.

RAVOLI WITH SPINACH

1 pkg. Mini Ravioli stuffed with prosciutto
1 pkg. Fresh Spinach
Salt to taste
1 T. Olive Oil
4 cloves Garlic peeled
Reggiano Parmigiana Cheese

Cook ravioli according to directions on package. Wash spinach. In a skillet add olive oil and garlic. Sauté for a minute. Add spinach, quarter glass of water, and salt. Cover skillet. Simmer for 2 minutes or until spinach wilts. Strain ravioli and add to spinach. Toss. Top with cheese. Serve.

SALMON CAKES

1 lb. Salmon Fillets
1 c. Bread Crumbs
¼ c. Light Cream
1 T. Mayonnaise
1 T. Worcestershire Sauce
2 T. Parsley
1 T. Baking Soda
Salt and Pepper to taste
¼ tsp. Garlic Powder
2 Eggs
1 qt. Vegetable Oil
2 T. Vinegar

In a pan, poach salmon in a bath of water with vinegar until it turns pink. Strain, cool, and crumble. In a bowl add salmon, bread crumbs, cream, mayonnaise, Worcestershire sauce, parsley, baking soda, salt, pepper, garlic powder, and eggs. Mix with hands until all ingredients are well blended. Preheat vegetable oil in a skillet. Take a tablespoonful of mixture and flatten with hand to form a pattie. Place into heated oil and when one side is golden brown, turn. Once both sides are golden brown place onto paper towels to absorb excess oil. Serve.

SAUSAGE AND POTATOES

4 Sausage links
4 Potatoes
Olive Oil

Poke holes into sausage links and place in a warm pan on top of stove. Cook until brown on all sides. Wash, peel and slice potatoes. Place in same pan as sausage. Cover and cook until potatoe is cook to desired tenderness. Serve.

SAUSAGE, GNOCCHI, AND MUSHROOMS

2 Sausage links
5 sliced Mushrooms
1 T. Parsley
1 T. Butter

1 batch Gnocchi (see recipe pg 53). Strain cooked gnocchi. Cut up sausage and brown in a skillet. Strain excess liquid. Add butter and mushrooms. Simmer for 3 minutes. Add parsley, and gnocchi. Toss. Serve.

SLOPPY TACO CHIPS

2 c. Tortilla Chips
1 lb. Chopped Meat
1 c. Iceberg Lettuce chopped
1 c. Tomatoes chopped
¼ c. Onion peeled and chopped
½ c. Cheddar Cheese shredded
¼ c. Black Olives chopped
3 T. Sour Cream
3 T. Taco or Salsa Sauce

In a pan, brown chopped meat. Strain. Place tortilla chips on a platter. Add cooked chopped meat on top of tortilla chips. Then add cheddar cheese, tomatoes, onion, olives, lettuce, taco or salsa sauce, and sour cream. Serve.

ONE PAN TURKEY DINNER

½ c. Gravy
1 c. Turkey shredded
½ c. leftover Stuffing

In a sauce pan heat gravy. Once it starts to bubble lower heat and add turkey. Simmer for 2 minutes. Add stuffing and simmer for another 2 minutes. Serve.

BAKED ZITI ON A PLATTER

½ lb. Ziti Pasta
¼ c. Ricotta
1 tsp. Grated Cheese
¼ c. Mozzarella shredded
1 c. Tomatoe sauce

Cook pasta according to package directions. Strain. Heat tomatoe sauce in a skillet. On a platter add macaroni, ricotta, grated cheese, mozzarella, and tomatoe sauce. Toss and serve.

A LOT OF SANDWICH

¼ lb. Ham
¼ lb. Salami
¼ lb. Provolone Cheese
1 loaf Crusty Bread
¼ head Iceberg Lettuce
¼ Onion
1 Tomatoe
1 T. Olive Oil
1 tsp. Oregano
1 tsp. Vinegar
Dash Salt

Wash and chop lettuce, and tomatoe. Peel and chop onion. Place in a bowl. Add olive oil, vinegar, oregano, and salt. Toss. Cut crusty bread lengthwise. Place ham, salami, cheese on one side. Spoon lettuce mixture on the other side. Pour remaining liquid on top of lettuce mixture. Fold together and slice into small sections. Serve.

_____

_____

_____

_____

TAC N' EGGS

¼ c. Salsa
½ lb. Chopped Meat
½ c. Iceberg Lettuce chopped
¼ c. Tomatoes chopped
¼ c. Onion peeled and chopped
½ c. Cheddar Cheese shredded
¼ c. Black Olives chopped
2 T. Sour Cream
2 Eggs
1 T. Butter
Tortilla Wraps

In a saucepan brown chopped meat. Strain. In a bowl beat eggs. In another pan melt butter and add eggs. Mix until cooked. On a platter place tortilla wraps and layer cooked chopped meat, salsa, scrambled eggs, lettuce, onion, cheddar cheese, olives, sour cream. Roll up and serve.

TORTELLINI WITH PEAS

1 pkg. Frozen Tortellini
1 pkg. Frozen Peas
1 tsp. Butter
1 pinch Pepper

Cook tortellini according to directions on package. At the last minute of cooking tortellini add frozen peas. Strain. In a bowl add tortellini, peas, butter, and pepper. Serve.

TURKEY POT PIES

1 c. Gravy
2 slices Turkey
¼ c. Mixed Vegetables strained
1 c. Stuffing leftover

Preheat broiler. Heat gravy in a saucepan that can go into the oven. Shred and add turkey to gravy. Add mixed vegetables and let simmer for 2 minutes. Place stuffing on top of gravy, turkey, and mixed vegetables. Place under broiler for 3 minutes or until the stuffing gets a crusty golden brown. Serve.

TURKEY SANDWICH

1 Bread Roll
2 slices Turkey
1 heaping Stuffing leftover
1 slice Cranberry Sauce
¼ c. Gravy

Heat up gravy in a saucepan. Slice roll and toast under broiler. Place turkey, stuffing, cranberry sauce, and drizzle gravy on toasted roll. Serve.

ZUCCHINI FRITTATA

2 Zucchini's chopped
1 clove Garlic
½ Onion peeled and chopped
3 Eggs
¼ c. Milk
2 T. Olive Oil
Salt and Pepper to taste

Preheat broiler. In a pan that can go into the oven place olive oil, onion, and garlic. Cook on low heat until onion softens. Add zucchini, salt, and pepper. In a bowl beat eggs and milk. Add to pan with olive oil, onion, garlic, and zucchini. Cook for 10 minutes on low heat. Place under broiler for another 5 minutes or until top turns golden brown. Serve with crusty bread.

GARLIC BREAD

1 loaf Italian Bread
2 T. Olive Oil
2 cloves Garlic peeled and chopped

Preheat oven to 350 degrees. On a long piece of aluminum foil, make slices on the loaf of bread half way down to the bottom. In between each slice sprinkle olive oil and chopped garlic. Wrap the loaf of bread up with the aluminum foil and place in the oven for 10 minutes. Unwrap loaf and serve.

TOASTED ITALIAN BREAD

1 loaf Italian Bread
1 T. Olive Oil
1 clove Garlic peeled and chopped
1 tsp. Red Pepper Flakes
1 tsp. Basil
1 tsp. Oregano
1 T. Grated Cheese

Preheat oven to 350 degrees. Slice Italian bread lengthwise in half and put in oven until golden brown about 2 minutes each side. Mix olive oil, garlic, red pepper flakes, basil, oregano, and grated cheese in a bowl. Place mixture on top of toasted bread. Place back into oven for another minute. Serve.

BANANA SPLIT WITH THE WORKS

1 Banana
1 scoop Vanilla Ice Cream
1 scoop Chocolate Ice Cream
¼ c. Pineapples in heavy syrup
2 T. Marshmallow Sauce
2 T. Chocolate Syrup
2 T. Walnuts in Syrup
Whipped Cream
Cherries

Peel and slice banana, place in a bowl. Add ice cream on top of banana. Top ice cream with pineapples, marshmallow sauce, chocolate sauce, and walnuts. Add whipped cream and cherries. Serve.

CHALLA BREAD PUDDING

3 Eggs
6 Egg Yolks
5 c. Whole Milk
¼ c. Heavy Cream
1 ½ c. Sugar
1 ½ tsp. Vanilla
1 tsp Cinnamon
1 loaf Challa Bread
1 c. Raisins

Preheat oven to 350 degrees. In a large bowl whisk the whole eggs, yolks, milk, heavy cream, sugar, vanilla and cinnamon. Set mixture aside. In a baking dish crumble half loaf of the challa bread. Sprinkle raisins on top. Crumble remaining half loaf of the challa bread. Pour mixture on top. Press down occasionally for 10 minutes. Place baking dish in a large pan with water about half way up the dish. Place a piece of aluminum foil on top of dish to form a tent. Cut some holes in the foil. Bake for 45 minutes. Remove from the oven and cool. Serve warm or at room temperature.

CHOCOLATE CREAM PIE

15 Marshmallows
1 4oz. bar Chocolate
½ c. Milk
1 pt. Heavy Cream
2 tsp. Vanilla
1 Graham Cracker Pie Crust
2 tsp. Sugar
1 tsp. Cinnamon
Grinded Roasted Almonds

Place marshmallows, milk, and chocolate bar in a double boiler under low heat, stir until melted. Let cool. In another bowl add ¼ cup of the heavy cream, one teaspoon sugar, cinnamon, one teaspoon vanilla and whip. Fold into cooled mixture. Pour into pie shell. Refrigerate. Once refrigerated, whip remaining heavy cream, vanilla, and sugar. Place on top of pie. Sprinkle roasted almonds on top. Serve.

HONEY BALLS

2 c. Flour
3 Eggs
1 T. Olive Oil
1 Lemon Skin grated
1 T. Sugar
2 T. Vanilla
½ tsp. Baking Powder
2 c. Vegetable Oil
½ c. Honey
Candied Sprinkles

Mix flour, eggs, olive oil, grated lemon skin, sugar, vanilla, baking powder in a bowl until a ball forms. Place oil in a pan and heat. Cut strips of dough. Roll between hands until a log is formed. Slice log into small pieces and roll pieces into balls. Drop into heated oil carefully. Once golden on all sides, take out of oil and place onto paper towels to drain excess oil. Then place in a bowl. Pour honey and mix all over balls. Add candied sprinkles and mix again. Serve.

ICE BOX CAKE

1 box Graham Crackers
1 16oz. container Chocolate Pudding
Whipped Cream

In a glass dish place one layer of graham crackers. Top with 2 tablespoons of chocolate pudding. Continue with another layer of graham crackers and chocolate pudding. Keep layering until you reach the rim of the dish. End with chocolate pudding. Crumble one or two graham crackers. Place crumbs on top of chocolate pudding. Refrigerate for 3 hours or overnight. Slice ice box cake and serve with whipped cream.

POUND CAKE DELIGHT

1 Pound Cake sliced
Whipped Cream
Drizzle of Chocolate Syrup

Put one piece of pound cake on a plate and top with whipped cream. Continue layering slices of pound cake and whipped cream until finished. End with whipped cream. Drizzle chocolate syrup on top. Serve.

PUMPKIN PIE

1 Pumpkin about 1 lb.
1 12oz. can Evaporated Milk
½ c. Sugar
¼ c. Brown Sugar
½ tsp. Ginger
½ tsp. Salt
1 tsp. Cinnamon
2 Eggs
2 Unbaked Pie Shells
Whipped Cream

Preheat oven to 325 degrees. Peel pumpkin and cut into chunks. Place on a cookie sheet and bake for 1 hour and 20 minutes. Pumpkin is done when fork goes through to bottom of pumpkin chunk. Strain pumpkin. Let cool. In blender, add 2 cups of pumpkin, evaporated milk, sugars, ginger, salt, cinnamon, and eggs. Preheat oven to 425 degrees. Poke holes with a fork into bottom of unbaked pie shells. Place in oven for 2 minutes. Pour pumpkin mixture into pie shells and bake in oven at 425 degrees for 15 minutes. Reduce heat to 350 degrees and bake for 45 minutes longer. Serve warm or cold with whipped cream.

RICOTTA CHEESE PLUS

¼ c. Ricotta Cheese
1 Chocolate Covered Strawberry
1 tsp. Honey

Place ricotta cheese in a dish. Quarter chocolate covered strawberry. Add on top of cheese. Drizzle honey all over. Serve.

STRAWBERRY SHORTCAKE

3 slices Pound Cake
Whipped Cream
4 sliced Strawberries
1 tsp. Chocolate Syrup

Place one slice of pound cake on a plate. Add some slices of strawberries and top with whipped cream. Repeat until all ingredients are finished. End with top layer of whipped cream. Drizzle with chocolate syrup. Serve.

STRAWBERRY TREAT

1 pt. Strawberries
1 tsp. Sugar
4 scoops Vanilla Ice Cream

Wash, hull and slice strawberries in a bowl. Add sugar. Let sit for 1 hour. Place strawberry mixture into a blender. Blend for a few seconds. Pour some of the liquid in a glass. Add a scoop of vanilla ice cream. Repeat layers. Serve with a straw and spoon.

CRUMBLED CHOCOLATE LAYERED TREAT

1 box Chocolate Cake Mix
Whipped Cream
1 jar Caramel Sauce
1 jar Cherries

Bake chocolate cake according to directions. Let cool. Crumble cake. Layer the bottom of a bowl with some chocolate crumbled cake. Next spread some whipped cream on top of the chocolate crumbled cake. Drizzle caramel sauce on top of the whipped cream. Continue layering until you reach the top of the bowl. End the top layer with whipped cream. Place the cherries on the top and drizzle some of the juice from the cherries onto the whipped cream. When serving scoop from the bottom up.

CREAM PUFFS

½ pint Heavy Cream
½ pint Milk
1 env. Dream Whip
1 box instant Vanilla Pudding Mix

1 stick Margarine
1 c. Boiled Water
¼ tsp. Salt
1 c. Flour
4 Eggs
1 tsp. Vanilla Extract

In a large bowl, add heavy cream, milk, dream whip, instant vanilla pudding mix and beat until thick and smooth. Refrigerate.

In a pot, bring boiled water and margarine to a second boil. Once margarine has melted, stir in flour and salt with a wooden spoon. Stir fast, until mixture leaves the side of pot and forms a dough like consistency. Remove from heat for 1 minute. In the same pot, with a wooden spoon beat in eggs, one at a time until smooth and doughy. Last add vanilla extract. Mix into dough. Preheat oven to 400 degrees. On a non-stick cookie sheet place a wooden spoonful of mixture to form three in a row about 1 inch in between each spoonful. Bake for 13 minutes. Lower oven to 350 degrees and bake for another 18 minutes. Let puffs cool completely. Slice in half lengthwise. Fill with 1 tablespoon of cream mixture. Refrigerate. Serve cold.

TRIPLE LAYER TREAT

3 Chocolate Chip Cookies
3 Scoops Vanilla Ice Cream
3 T. Whipped Cream
Chopped Nuts

Crumble cookies. Divide into three piles. In a glass, place one pile of crumbs on bottom followed by one scoop ice cream, a tablespoon of whipped cream, sprinkle of chopped nuts. Repeat layer two more times. Serve.

CANDY CLUSTER

¼ c. Raisins
¼ c. Walnuts, Almonds or Hazelnuts
¼ c. Coconut shredded
2 large bars Chocolate

In a double boiler, melt chocolate. Once chocolate has melted add raisins, nuts, and coconut. Take a wooded spoonful of mixture and place onto some wax paper. Let cool. Serve.

CHOCOLATE COVERED STRAWBERRIES

1 11oz. Milk Chocolate Morsels
2 lbs. Long Stem Strawberries

Place morsels in a double boiler and melt. Stir with wooden spoon. Wash strawberries and dry completely. Dip strawberries into melted chocolate. Place onto waxed paper. Refrigerate until chocolate hardens. Serve.

CHOCOLATE SANDWICH COOKIES

1 log Sugar Cookie Dough
1 16oz. bar Milk Chocolate
Candied Sprinkles
Crushed Nuts

Preheat oven to 350 degrees. Slice cookie dough and place on cookie sheet. Bake for 16 minutes. Let cool. In a double boiler melt chocolate bar. Dip cooled cookies into melted chocolate. Place onto waxed paper. Sprinkle with candied sprinkles and/or crushed nuts. Let cool. Serve.

KNOTS

6 Eggs
1 c. Sugar
1 c. Oil
2 tsp. Vanilla Extract
5 c. Flour
5 tsp. Baking Powder
1 pinch Salt
1 Orange peel grated
¼ c. Confectionery Sugar
2 drops Water
Food Coloring
1 drop Almond Extract

Preheat oven to 350 degrees. Mix eggs, sugar, oil, vanilla, flour, baking powder, salt, and grated orange peel in a bowl to form a dough. Cut small pieces and roll between hands into a small log. Take the two ends and tie into a knot. Place onto cookie sheet. Bake 15-20 minutes. Let cool. Mix confectionery sugar, water, food coloring, and almond extract in a dish. Dip top of knot into mixture. Place on a rack until icing dries. Serve.

SUGAR MINT CHOCOLATE COOKIES

1 log Sugar Dough Cookie
1 bar Mint Chocolate Candy

Preheat oven to 350 degrees. Slice cookie dough and place on cookie sheet. Crumble mint chocolate candy bar and place some pieces on top of each slice of cookie dough. Bake 16 minutes. Cool and serve.

CRANBERRY ORANGE RELISH

1 bag Fresh Cranberries
1 Orange
1 tsp. Grated Orange Peel
½ c. Sugar

Grate Orange. Slice Orange. Combine cranberries, orange, orange peel, and sugar into a food processor. Pulse two or three times. Refrigerate and serve chilled.

HONEY MUSTARD SAUCE

1 T. Honey
2 T. Mustard

In a bowl mix honey and mustard together until blended.
Serve.

TARTAR SAUCE

½ c. Mayonnaise
½ c. Onion peeled and chopped
½ Lemon
Pinch Salt and Pepper
1 clove Garlic minced
1 c. Sweet Pickles chopped

Combine mayonnaise, onion, lemon, salt, pepper, garlic, sweet pickles in a food processor. Pulse two or three times. Transfer to a bowl and refrigerate for an hour. Serve chilled.

Give flowers to someone you do not know.

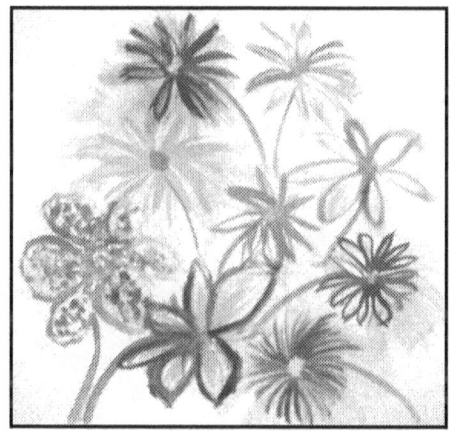

For more information about the author and the book
please go to:

msrega@comcast.net

www.trafford.com/06-1976